AF290325

THE SECRETS OF BETTER SLEEP

Get a great night's sleep,
every night!

Written by Vera Smayan
In collaboration with Céline Faidherbe
Translated by Rebecca Neal

Health and Wellbeing 50MINUTES.com

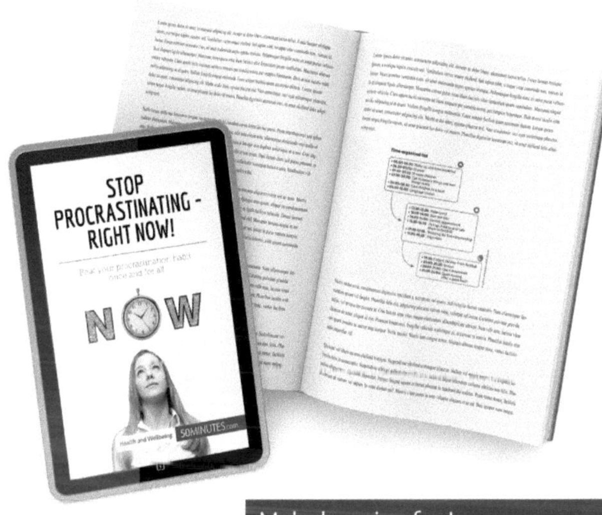

THE SECRETS OF BETTER SLEEP

GET A GREAT NIGHT'S SLEEP, EVERY NIGHT!

- **Problem:** getting enough good-quality sleep is essential for our overall quality of life, but this is not always easy. Nowadays, many adults are looking for ways to improve their sleeping habits.
- **Aim:** to better understand sleep and its importance, to learn about the most common sleep problems, and to discover good habits, tips and alternative therapies to get a great night's rest.
- **FAQs:**
  - Is it correct to say that we sleep to rest?
  - Do our genes determine the amount of sleep we need?
  - Is sleepwalking a sleep disorder?
  - Is it true that the older we get, the less sleep we need?
  - Is it true that any sleep we get before mid-

night is twice as restful?
  ◦ What is the optimal sleeping position?
  ◦ Am I doing the right thing by following seve-
    ral different treatments to cure my sleeping
    problems?

Since time immemorial, sleep has been both an essential component of life and a fascinating enigma, as can be seen in the famous lines from Shakespeare's (English playwright, 1564-1616) play *The Tempest*: "We are such stuff/As dreams are made on, and our little life/Is rounded with a sleep" (Act IV, Scene I).

Indeed, we spend a significant proportion of our time sleeping – most of us will spend around a third of our lives asleep. Getting plenty of good-quality sleep is crucial to our wellbeing, while sleep deprivation can lead to a host of physical and mental health problems.

But what really happens when we are asleep? Even today, we do not have all the answers to this question. Although studies over the past hundred years or so have shed some light on the mysteries of sleep, their results are only the tip of the iceberg.

In our increasingly fast-paced society, it can be easy to forget that sleep is a natural part of life and a crucial factor in our recovery from tiredness and the efforts of our day-to-day lives. However, a good night's sleep has become something of a luxury, because it requires us to maintain a consistent daily schedule and respect our body clock. Consequently, nowadays a significant proportion of the population suffers from sleep deprivation and/or poor sleep quality.

In under 50 minutes, you will learn how sleep works and discover natural ways of achieving good-quality rest. By respecting your physical and mental needs, developing good habits and preserving your body's natural rhythms, you can find a sleep schedule that works for you and lets you wake up feeling refreshed and ready to take on the day ahead.

WHAT IS SLEEP?

Sleep is a heterogenous physiological state that affects the entire body. It is characterised by a range of changes in the body's functioning and, most importantly, by the temporary suspension of consciousness and alertness, which are always present when we are awake. It plays an essential role in our body's homeostasis (the maintenance of equilibrium in our functions).

Sleep is a period of rest which is distinct from our waking hours, as our conscious mind shuts off and our body's energy is restored. Sleep is therefore a time for both physical and mental recovery characterised by the temporary absence of our consciousness and will, the slowing of the functions of our nervous system and the partial interruption of our sensory and motor relationships with our environment. Our bodies cannot fully relax and recover without sleep.

Over the centuries, sleep has been contrasted with wakefulness, which is linked to consciousness and reality. However, the Vedas, a body of ancient Indian texts dating from the 12th century BCE, outline an alternative perspective which does not view sleep as the antithesis of wakefulness, but rather as an alternative state of consciousness. Indeed, when we dream, our bodily functions are as active as they are during our waking hours, and our mental experiences at these times are no less real simply because they occur while we are asleep. What we call "reality" is merely a matter of perception, which is determined by our brain activity. In fact, the Vedas outline four different states of consciousness: waking, dreaming, deep sleep (meaning sleep without dreams) and turiya, a state of pure consciousness that serves as an omnipresent background to the other three states.

In Greek mythology, Morpheus (the son of Hypnos, the god of sleep, and Nyx, the goddess of the night) is the god of dreams and tries to make mortals fall asleep. He is often depicted as a young man with a mirror in one hand and poppies, which cause drowsiness, in the other. He also has wings like a butterfly's, which flutter silently. He makes people fall asleep by touching them with poppies, and morphine (which is derived from poppies) takes its name from him. Many languages use expressions like "in the arms of Morpheus" to refer to someone who is in a deep, calm sleep.

Scientists, artists and philosophers from all over the world have long been interested in sleep, as this alternative state of existence raises an endless list of questions about human perception, how our brains work and the nature of reality.

SLEEP CYCLES

Sleep is made up of cycles of around one and a half to two hours that follow on from one another.

Consequently, in the course of a night we will go through several sleep cycles of varying lengths. Each cycle ends with a transitional phase (sometimes accompanied by a brief period of wakefulness) leading into a new cycle.

These cycles comprise two types of sleep: slow-wave sleep and rapid eye movement sleep (REM).

- In adults, a phase of slow-wave sleep lasts for around 75 minutes and comprises four sub-states of increasingly deep sleep. This type of sleep accounts for almost 80% of our night.
- Slow-wave sleep is followed by a phase of REM sleep, so called because it is characterised by rapid random movement of the eyes. This phase lasts for around 20 minutes and is the time when our brains are most active. It is believed that dreams occur during REM sleep.

In general, we go through four or five cycles each time we sleep, and the length of each type of sleep differs between cycles. Specifically, the first cycle features a particularly long and intense phase of slow-wave sleep and a short period of REM sleep, and this proportion is gradually reversed in subsequent cycles.

Sleep cycles

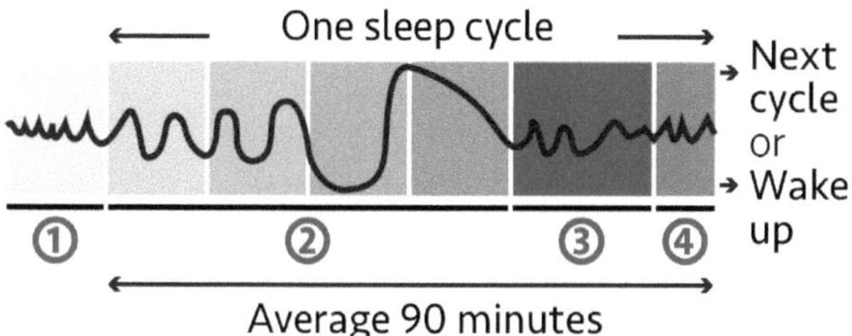

Each sleep cycle comprises the following phases:

- **phase I:** very light sleep (moment of falling asleep);
- **phase II:** light slow-wave sleep;
- **phase III:** deep slow-wave sleep;
- **phase IV:** very deep slow-wave sleep;
- **REM phase.**

Phases III and IV have the greatest effect on our recovery. It has been proven that our bodies recover best during the first hours of sleep, when there is a greater proportion of deep sleep, no matter whether we go to bed before midnight or in the early hours of the morning.

At the end of phase IV, we transition into REM sleep, when we tend to dream more vividly. REM sleep is also sometimes known as para-doxical sleep because, although it is a phase of deep sleep, our brain activity is similar to when we are awake and the physiological functions controlled by the central nervous system are fully active. Our breathing is irregular, our blood pressure increases, and we experience feelings and sensations. Consequently, although we are still asleep, our physiological state is very similar to when we are awake.

Sometimes, the border between sleep and wakefulness becomes blurred. During prolonged periods of sleep deprivation (known as "sleep debt", meaning the cumulative effect of not get-ting enough sleep), a person who is awake may experience brief moments where they are not fully conscious, and during which they can even dream and hallucinate.

THE STATES OF SLEEP

The criteria used to define the states of sleep are based on the activity recorded though EEG (electroencephalography) on the surface of the skull under laboratory conditions. This has allowed scientists to study the conditions at the beginning of, during and at the end of sleep, and in particular the neurological and physiological mechanisms that are responsible for these states.

When we are sleeping, our bodies undergo significant muscular, hormonal, metabolic and behavioural changes. The functions of the automatic nervous system, such as blood pressure and digestion, speed up or slow down depending on the phase of sleep, and conscious mental activity (state of alertness) is suspended.

During slow-wave sleep, the electrical waves in our brain slow down, going from alpha waves in phase I, when we are sleeping lightly, to delta waves in phase IV, the period of deep sleep that is followed by REM sleep.

<u>SHORT AND LONG SLEEPERS</u>

If you go to bed after 11pm and only need six hours of sleep or less to wake up feeling refreshed, you are what is known as a short sleeper.

The amount of sleep you need is not a reflection on you as a person: our sleep needs are determined by our genes. This means that so-called long sleepers need nine or ten hours of sleep to recover adequately, and sleeping less than this will negatively impact their wellbeing.

The average person needs six to eight hours of sleep per night. To remain in good physical and mental shape, you need to respect your body's own sleep needs, which will not necessarily be the same as other people's.

THE IMPORTANCE OF GOOD-QUALITY SLEEP

However, the precise physiological role of sleep remains shrouded in mystery. Although sleep appears to be a state of complete calm, it is also a time when complex changes take place in our brains, which cannot be fully explained by the hypothesis that sleep is a time of physical and mental rest. In fact, the activity levels of some brain cells during certain phases of sleep are five to ten times higher than when we are awake!

One thing, at least, is clear: sleep plays a fundamental role in repair and regeneration. For example, it helps to develop our memories and immune responses, and stimulates functions that are essential to the regulation of our bodies, including protein synthesis, tissue repair, the working of muscle cells and toxin elimination.

Sleep deprivation and poor-quality sleep both have negative effects on our health and quality of life. Specifically, they typically result in a feeling of tiredness and drowsiness (the leading cause of car accidents), impaired cognitive function, a disrupted metabolism and a weakened immune system, as well as an increased risk of obesity and cardiovascular disease.

Lack of sleep also has serious consequences on our mental health: it can lead to irritability, anxiety and even depression. Indeed, sleep deprivation is a contributing factor to a range of psychiatric disorders.

SLEEP DISORDERS

Sleep disorders refer to any disturbance in the length or quality of our sleep. They can be divided into three main categories: dyssomnias (reduced quality and quantity of sleep), hypersomnia (too much sleep) and parasomnias (abnormal behaviour during sleep).

Sleep disorders can be caused by a range of factors, including anxiety, depression, apnoea and distractions in the sufferer's environment. The real problem is the fact that sleep disorders can result in a vicious circle that is hard to break. A person who is anxious about sleeping well is likely to make poor dietary choices, further damaging the quality of their sleep. This makes them even more anxious about getting a good night's sleep, and their sleep quality deteriorates even further.

As a general rule, the primary cause of most sleep disorders can be found in our modern lifestyles, as we often find ourselves in a state of hypervigilance and stress which disturbs our natural biological rhythms.

INSOMNIA

Insomnia is without a doubt the most common sleep disorder, affecting between 15 and 20% of adults in Western countries. However, not all cases of insomnia are equal: there is a difference between chronic insomnia, which is fortunately quite rare, and temporary insomnia, in which sufferers only occasionally struggle to fall asleep or end up waking frequently in the night.

There are two kinds of insomnia: primary insomnia, which has no external cause, and secondary insomnia, which is a side effect of another illness or other circumstances.

SLEEPING PATTERNS THROUGHOUT HISTORY

Historical accounts and scientific evidence have shown that our ancestors never slept for eight hours in one go, even though nowadays this is held up as the standard for healthy sleeping patterns.

According to a 2001 study by Roger Ekirch, a historian at Virginia Tech University, until the 18th century humans slept in two phases rather than one: in other words, our ancestors woke up in the middle of the night to reflect, work or even visit neighbours, among other activities, before going back to bed. They would typically sleep for three or four hours, wake up for an hour or so, then go back to sleep until morning.

Further evidence for this hypothesis comes from tests carried out by Thomas Wehr of the National Institute of Mental Health in the 1990s, which demonstrated that biphasic sleep comes naturally to humans. This means that we naturally wake up at the quietest, calmest period of the night and go back to sleep a few hours later. Even today, monks in a number of religions use this time to pray and meditate.

RESTLESS LEGS SYNDROME (RLS)

The main symptoms of RLS are movement, pins and needles and pain in the legs. Immobility exacerbates these symptoms, which means that they are worse in the evening and at night. It is an intermittent problem: sufferers generally report alternating periods of severe and mild symptoms.

The causes of RLS have still not been conclusively identified, although researchers are currently looking into a potential link between the disorder and iron or magnesium deficiencies, disruptions in dopamine production, or diabetes.

OBSTRUCTIVE SLEEP APNOEA (OSA)

The severity of OSA varies between sufferers. It is characterised by momentary interruptions to breathing during sleep, which can occur anywhere from five to 30 times per hour.

Sufferers are generally not aware of the problem until they are told by someone else, who has noticed that they stop breathing while they are asleep. Many OSA sufferers are drowsy during the day, because the momentary interruptions to their sleep prevent them from resting properly, meaning that they wake up feeling tired. Other signs of the problem include snoring, night sweats, a dry mouth and saliva on the pillow.

OSA mainly affects older or obese individuals. It can have serious consequences for sufferers' health, namely disturbances in the neuroendocrine system (which makes the individual more prone to weight gain, hormone disorders, cardiovascular disease and diabetes, among other health problems), memory problems, irritability and depression.

SLEEPWALKING

As the name suggests, sleepwalkers get up and move around at night while they are unconscious, during deep slow-wave sleep. It is linked to problems in the thalamus and cortex, which are responsible for the transition between sleep and wakefulness and the disconnection of the brain from sensory stimulation during deep sleep. Each episode of sleepwalking can last for up to 30 minutes.

Sleepwalking is not generally dangerous because most people only carry out simple, everyday activities such as sitting on their bed or going to the bathroom. However, in more severe cases, the sleepwalker may become violent or perform dangerous activities such as driving.

THE KEYS TO GOOD-QUALITY SLEEP

A HEALTHY LIFESTYLE

There are a wide range of natural remedies and holistic therapies (meaning those which treat the person as a whole rather than focusing on a specific problem) which can be very useful in treating sleep disorders.

All sleep problems, whether they are a cause or a consequence of a sleep disorder, disturb our circadian rhythm, meaning the rhythm of the body's functions over a period of roughly 24 hours. The circadian rhythm is regulated by cues such as light, which marks the shift from day to night.

GO TO BED AT THE RIGHT TIME

The best time to go to bed is when you start to feel drowsy, which obviously differs from one person to another. Drowsiness occurs at regular intervals of between 90 and 130 minutes. Pay close attention to the first signs of tiredness, because if you stay awake past them, it will be a while until the optimal moment for sleep comes around again.

Your first priority should therefore be to adjust your lifestyle to find mental and physical balance. In this section, we will outline some general suggestions and recommendations to help you achieve this.

Light and melatonin production

Light plays a crucial role in the regulation of sleep and wakefulness. The presence of light is detected by our eyes and then communicated to our central nervous system, which stimulates the production of melatonin, the hormone that regulates sleep, in the pineal gland. Melatonin production begins in the evening and decreases over the course of the night until we wake up. As well as sleep, this hormone also influences our appetite, libido and immune system. After we reach the age of 50, we begin to produce less melatonin, which partly explains why older people tend to have more trouble falling asleep.

The light we are exposed to in our everyday lives can seriously disturb our sleep. The wavelengths of the blue light given off by devices such as tablets and computers (450-480 nanometres) delay melatonin synthesis and encourage us to stay awake. Studies have shown that half an hour of exposure to blue light between 11pm and 1am is enough to confuse our body clock.

The following simple precautions can help you to avoid the harmful effects of blue light:

- switch off electronic devices and stay away from screens giving off blue light for at least two hours before going to bed;
- remember that exposure to light and exercise outdoors during the day are vital, as this will allow your body to regulate its sleep-wake rhythm;
- if necessary, and with the supervision of a doctor, take melatonin capsules to make up for a deficiency in production.

On the other hand, the overproduction of melatonin during winter is believed to be one of the causes of tiredness and seasonal depression.

One recommended method for dealing with melatonin deficiency is light therapy, which involves using a special lamp to increase your exposure to light. Light therapy is also an effective way of resetting your body clock after a long trip.

You can buy lamps which give off between 2500 and 10 000 lux (the unit used to measure light) to put on your desk for half an hour every morning, or follow a treatment course at a specialised light therapy centre.

The benefits of naps

Naps, meaning brief periods of light sleep, have a range of health benefits as they allow us to partially catch up on a sleep debt accumulated over a period of several days. Ideally, you should sleep for 20 minutes between 1pm and 3pm, and make sure that you do not sleep for more than 40 minutes, as this could affect your sleep that night.

For a long time, naps were an accepted part of everyday life. However, with the increased pace of our everyday lives, they are increasingly seen as a waste of valuable time and have become less common. Many people still take regular naps in southern European countries, where it is harder to resist a short nap after a heavy lunch, particular if the weather is hot.

We are biologically hardwired to sleep at the start of the afternoon, regardless of whether or not we have eaten a good meal. Our circadian rhythm dictates that our need for sleep is more intense between 1am and 5am, and between 2pm and 4pm. Naps therefore have benefits for individuals and for society as whole. If it is possible for you to work a nap into your daily schedule, this will help you to return to a healthier, more natural sleep-wake rhythm.

The importance of diet

Although many of us tend to neglect our diet, it is essential to our overall health and to good sleep. Eating food that is too rich in the evening can damage the quality of our sleep, while not eating enough may cause us to wake up because we are hungry.

The more you weigh, the more likely you are to suffer from sleep disorders, as excess weight can cause breathing problems and snoring during the night.

It is therefore essential to eat a balanced diet and follow a few basic rules.

- Eat your evening meal at around 8pm, and at least two hours before going to bed.
- Eat a good-sized portion of light food to avoid waking up in the night.
- Avoid drinks containing caffeine after 5pm.

It is also important to regularly consume foods containing magnesium, as this helps to regulate the nervous system, especially if it is ingested alongside vitamin B6. Good sources of magnesium and vitamin B6 include green leafy vegetables, spinach, almonds, walnuts and cereals.

Foods to encourage sleep

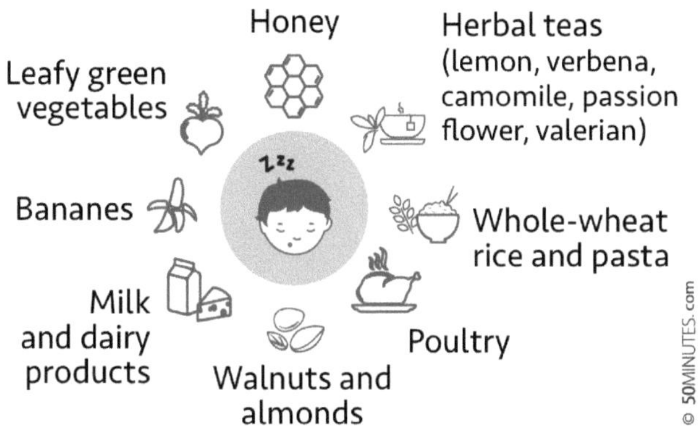

Conversely, foods that are high in vitamin C (such as oranges, lemons and grapefruit), legumes, fried foods, sauces, fishes and eggs should be avoided before bed.

An ideal meal would therefore be a light dish comprising whole-wheat rice or pasta, a small quantity of poultry, ham or another lean meat, and a lettuce-based salad. A good desert would be a piece of fresh fruit or a low-fat yoghurt.

Exercise

Regular physical activity is crucial to a good quality of life and high-quality sleep. Studies have shown that exercising for an hour to an hour and a half three times per week makes it easier to fall asleep, limits waking up during the night and increases the regularity of sleep cycles. However, exercising too late in the day (after 7pm) can damage the quality of your sleep.

BEDTIME RITUALS

Below are a few suggestions for simple rituals to get you ready for bed:

- take a hot bath with a teaspoon of almond oil and two drops of lavender essential oil;
- listen to half an hour of classical music;
- massage your feet or head;

- put a few drops of sweet orange or mandarin essential oil in a diffuser;
- settle down with a good book.

Conversely, it is not recommended to:

- watch violent or emotional films;
- use your computer, tablet or smartphone;
- listen to the news;
- get into a discussion (or worse, an argument).

Getting into a routine will also help you to go to bed at a similar time each night.

THE IDEAL BEDROOM

The bedroom is one of the most important rooms in any house. A tidy, well-appointed room is essential if you want to make sure you get enough high-quality sleep.

- Ideally, you should sleep in total darkness, especially between midnight and 3am (when the pineal gland, which produces melatonin, is at its most active).
- It is also a good idea to have a lamp on each side of the bed to create a softer, less direct light.

- The ideal bedroom temperature is around 18°C.
- The quality of your mattress is inextricably linked to the quality of your sleep. Natural bedding may seem expensive, but it is a worthwhile investment for your health and wellbeing. Synthetic fabrics generate static electricity, which interferes with your bodily functions, while natural materials such as linen, wool, sisal and natural latex favour heat transfer. Your bed should be adapted to your body: neither too hard nor soft, and fitted to your body shape.
- Make sure you ventilate the room for at least 20 minutes every day.
- Electromagnetic fields interfere with sleep, so make sure you do not sleep next to electronic devices such as your television or your computer, and unplug your Wi-Fi, mobile phone and wireless landline.
- Use a diffuser with a few drops of a calming essential oil such as lavender, camomile, vanilla or orange blossom.

The tips below draw on feng shui (a traditional Chinese art which involves harmonising the energy in our environment to boost our wellbeing), and should enable you to create a haven where you can easily relax.

- Ideally, the bedroom should be located at the back and on the right of the house.
- To generate a feeling of security, the head of the bed should be close to the wall without touching it (around 30 cm away) so as not to disturb the passage of chi (energy). Contrary to received wisdom, the bed can face in any direction.
- Make sure that you have space on each side of the bed and that the mattress does not touch the floor. This will allow chi to circulate freely.
- Do not position the bed underneath a window, a beam or shelves, because this can generate a feeling of anxiety and tends to sap the sleeper's energy.
- Do not have the head of the bed facing the door or the bathroom wall, and do not have the foot of the bed opposite the door or on its direct axis. This is known as the coffin position, and will drain you of your energy.
- Make sure that the entrance to the room is visible from the bed, as this fosters a sense of

security. However, putting the bed too close to the door will put the subconscious on guard.

- Opt for furniture with rounded edges; according to feng shui, corners give off negative energy.
- Similarly, avoid sharp corners by choosing oval-shaped mirrors, as this will prevent feelings of anxiety, and make sure that you cover any mirrors before going to bed.
- The layout of the room should ensure that energy can circulate freely and you feel a sense of security. Tidy away anything that reminds you of work (papers, folders, etc.) and avoid letting books and other items accumulate; one book on your bedside table is all you need to have out at any one time.
- Avoid overly strong colours, such as red, and overly dark colours, as they increase your energy and stimulate you rather than relaxing you. Light, muted tones will have a relaxing effect.
- Choose a lighter colour for the ceiling than for the walls, as a dark-coloured ceiling reduces the room's energy or results in stagnant energy.
- Make sure that your bed is made of wood,

with no metal parts. Feng shui works because it harmonises the room and balances the complementary concepts of yin and yang. This means that you need to avoid materials that are too "yang", meaning hard, smooth, cold materials such as marble and glass.

EMOTION AND STRESS LEVELS

Inner calm is essential for regular, good-quality sleep. However, this is often easier said than done...

We have all fallen into bed at the end of a long day, only to find that our brain starts whirring as soon as our head hits the pillow. No matter how tired we are, sleep seems out of reach. This situation is especially frustrating if we wake up in the middle of the night and cannot fall back to sleep until daybreak.

Learning to manage your emotions and respect your physical needs is therefore an essential step in getting back into good sleeping habits. There are a range of techniques, including yoga and meditation, that can help you to get in touch with your emotions and increase your awareness of your body. Unlike anxiety medication and sleeping pills, these natural solutions have no side effects and carry no risk of addiction.

Sophrology

Sophrology was developed in the 1960s by the Colombian psychiatrist Alfonso Caycedo (1932-2017), and aims to study the consciousness. It can be carried out in individual or group sessions.

The visualisation, relaxation and breathing exercises that make up sophrology allow individuals to anticipate situations that cause them anxiety and manage them positively. Sophrology can therefore provide a solution for a range of sleep problems. Just a few sessions should be enough to reduce the anxiety linked to going to bed, which is common in insomniacs, and to eliminate any potential stress that can arise and result in a vicious circle.

Sophrology can also be used to tackle the root causes of sleep problems, such as physical, mental or emotional imbalances, or an unhealthy lifestyle.

Yoga

Yoga, which originated in northern India as an ascetic and meditative practice, is an ancient discipline comprising a range of techniques to promote physical and mental wellbeing. The most commonly practiced kind of yoga in Western countries is hatha yoga, which is based primarily on physical exercises.

Yoga leaves practitioners feeling both alert and relaxed. However, it is not recommended to practice yoga at the end of the day, as this may increase your energy levels and disturb your sleep.

Meditation

Meditation can allow you to reach a state of profound peace when your mind is completely relaxed. Achieving mindfulness will in turn stimulate your vital energy and enable you to regain a sense of physical, mental and emotional balance.

Meditation is not a series of exercises but rather a state of being. However, there are different postures and breathing exercises that can help you to relax more fully.

Meditation in the evening

It is recommended to mediate for ten minutes in the evening, for example while sitting with your feet in a bowl of lukewarm water with a fistful of coarse salt (which symbolises the Earth).

Close your eyes and simply let your thoughts flow, without trying to hold onto them or push them away. Focus as much as possible on your breathing, but do not force it. When you are done, throw out the water and wash the bowl, which should only be used for your meditation.

After you have done it a few times, meditation will start to come more naturally to you and the experience will be even more relaxing.

Hypnosis

Hypnosis can be an effective treatment for a range of sleep problems, particularly when the "vicious circle" of sleep disturbance is causing anxiety. A few sessions should be enough to allow you to reach a state of autohypnosis, which will enable you to relax and prepare for sleep every evening.

Cat therapy

Petting a cat and listening to it purr is relaxing and soothing, and helps to lessen the burden of our thoughts and emotions. The benefits of a cat's purr have been scientifically proven: it can reduce anxiety and improve sleep quality in both cats and humans. This is because the frequency of its vibrations (20-140 hertz) has a positive effect on the human body: specifically, it relaxes the nervous system, lowers blood pressure and helps injuries and bones to heal more quickly.

Phytotherapy

There are a number of plants that can help to restore our body's natural rhythms. The best options for treating insomnia are plants with soporific properties and those that can regulate the nervous system, including in particular:

- passion flower, which can reduce palpitations and spasms:
- camomile, a well-known treatment for nerves, digestive problems and difficulty sleeping;
- *Alchemilla*, which can help with digestive problems;
- hawthorn, which is extremely effective for settling nerves before bed or after waking up in the night;
- verbena, which should be taken in small doses to limit the risk of nausea;
- lemon balm;
- lime;
- hops, which have a powerful calming effect;
- valerian, which is effective in severe cases of insomnia, but can lead to dependence (it is advised not to take it for more than ten days in a row).

The synergy between passion flower and valerian is particularly powerful and promotes deep sleep.

These plants can be taken as infusions, in capsule form or as a mother tincture (fresh plant extract). If your sleeping problems stem from seasonal depression, the best course of action is usually St John's wort capsules. In gemmotherapy, which uses embryonic plant tissue such as seeds or shoots, a tincture made of fig buds is a classic treatment for insomnia because it soothes the stomach, which is often irritated because of stress and insomnia, and in turn prevents the sufferer from sleeping, resulting in a vicious circle.

You should consult a professional (herbalist, phytotherapy expert, pharmacist or naturopath) to decide on the plants and dose to use because, although medicinal plants do not have serious side effects, they are not completely risk-free. For example, you may need to avoid certain plants because of how they interact with some medications.

Bach flower remedies

These are alcoholic macerations made from 38 types of flower, each of which is used to treat a particular character trait or emotional state.

They can be taken alongside all other kinds of medication, and three in particular are very effective for treating sleeping problems:

- Vervain is recommended for individuals who suffer from overstimulation or anxiety and who struggle to relax as a result;
- White Chestnut helps to restore inner peace, and is recommended for people whose worries prevent them from sleeping or who wake up in the middle of the night;
- Agrimony is recommended for people whose apparently happy exterior conceals anxiety, who struggle to fall asleep and who have restless sleep.

The most common method is to take three drops of the remedy underneath the tongue three times per day. However, for best results you should always consult a specialist, who can recommend a treatment tailored to your particular needs.

Aromatherapy

There are a number of essential oils that can help with sleeping difficulties.

- Ravintsara is particularly beneficial for nervous, introverted individuals who tend to overthink and overanalyse things. It is especially effective at treating sleep problems linked to exhaustion.
- True lavender, camomile and ylang-ylang have calming properties and are recommended for extroverted, outgoing people who struggle to sleep because of their strong emotions.
- Verbena, which is fragrant and has calming and sedative properties, is useful for impatient and irritable individuals.
- Finally, neroli oil is a very effective way of treating issues with the nervous system. It is particularly useful in the case of sleeping difficulties linked to emotional pain, especially when taken in conjunction with camomile.

The easiest and best way to take essential oils is to add a few drops to a diffuser and breathe in their scent. They can also be ingested orally, with a small amount of honey, or through the skin, depending on the oil and your individual circumstances.

Even though essential oils are natural products, you still need to take some precautions when using them. Specifically, some essential oils are toxic and cannot be ingested orally, while others can be irritating and even corrosive when applied to the skin. Furthermore, they should never be administered to children under three years of age. It is therefore crucial to follow the recommendations of an aromatherapist or pharmacist and to avoid home remedies, which can be extremely dangerous.

Homeopathy

Homeopathy can be a very effective treatment for sleep problems, but the approach needed will depend on your symptoms and personality. It is therefore essential to consult a trained homeopath before embarking on a course of homeopathic treatment.

That said, in cases of occasional insomnia, the following treatments can be effective:

- *Arnica montana* (three granules at 5 CH [a unit of homeopathic dilution] three times per day) in case of difficulty falling asleep because of unusual physical activity;
- *Coffea cruda* (three granules at 30 CH three times per day) when sleep is disturbed by an overactive mind;
- *Nux vomica* (three granules at 5 CH three times per day) when sleep is disturbed by anger or stomach irritation.

There are also homeopathic compounds which combine multiple remedies and can be purchased over the counter in most pharmacies.

Acupuncture

Acupuncture is an ancient science that first developed in China, and can be very effective in treating sleep problems. It involves stimulating precise zones of the skin which correspond to points on the meridians (energy lines through which vital energy flows).

According to acupuncture, all health problems are caused by an imbalance in the body's energy. Once the acupuncturist has identified the source of this imbalance, they will insert needles into precise points to restore balance. Given that each case of sleep trouble is different, each acupuncture session is unique.

GOLDEN NEEDLE THERAPY

Golden needle therapy is a specific form of acupuncture that originated in Tibetan medicine. It is a particularly effective way of treating sleep problems.

It involves inserting a 24-carat gold needle into a point known as Baihui (meaning "hundred meetings" in Chinese) situated on the governing vessel (Du-20) on the top of the head. Stimulating this point releases accumulated fatigue and resets the sleep-wake cycle.

Shiatsu

Massage is one of the most effective ways of eliminating physical and mental tension and preparing for sleep.

Shiatsu, a kind of therapeutic massage which originated in Japan, shares some similarities with acupuncture in that it is based on the principle of the balance of vital energy, which can be achieved by applying pressure to specific points on the meridians. The person receiving the massage remains fully clothed and lies down on a futon. Positive results can generally be observed after just one session, with a sense of relaxation and wellbeing which will improve sleep quality.

Ayurveda

Ayurveda is a kind of ancient Indian medicine which identifies three kinds of energy, known as *doshas*: *Vata* (air), *Pitta* (fire) and *Kapha* (water and earth). All three *doshas* are present in all organisms, but a person's predominant type of energy will determine their temperament and the lifestyle they need to adopt to optimise their health.

Problems with insomnia are generally linked to an imbalance in *Vata* energy, which is characterised by anxiety, nervousness and mental agitation.

This energy can be rebalanced by eating hot, well-cooked foods instead of raw or cold meals, opting for sweeter flavours and increasing your intake of carminatives (foods which facilitate the expulsion of intestinal gas and prevent its formation, such as cumin, fennel and cardamom) and aromatic plants such as basil and rosemary.

Conversely, vegetables from the nightshade family, such as potatoes, tomatoes, aubergines, green peppers and raw onions, are to be avoided.

Another effective way of rebalancing your energies and getting a good night's sleep is to go to bed early after giving yourself a massage (foot massages are particularly recommended) to help your body relax.

Finally, regular physical activity forms part of the ayurvedic lifestyle, as this will keep you feeling healthy and help you to sleep. People for whom *Pitta* or *Kapha* energy predominates should opt for sports such as jogging and swimming, while those whose main energy type is *Vata* are better suited to dance or yoga.

Osteopathy

This is a kind of alternative medicine which uses gentle manipulation of the body to rebalance its energy, and can work wonders for sleep disorders such as restless legs syndrome or sleep apnoea. Sessions last for around an hour and are delivered by a trained practitioner.

Cognitive behavioural therapy (CBT)

This is a short, scientifically proven treatment which aims to replace negative ideas and unsuitable behaviours with new thoughts and responses that are better suited to the real situation. It is delivered via individual or group sessions, and can be an effective way of identifying and correcting behaviours that impair sleep, as these are often a cause and/or consequence of insomnia.

FAQS

IS IT CORRECT TO SAY THAT WE SLEEP TO REST?

Yes and no. Our bodies need sleep to recover, but after a massage, for example, we can feel just as rested as if we had slept. Sleep also fulfils other functions, which scientists are yet to fully understand and explain.

DO OUR GENES DETERMINE THE AMOUNT OF SLEEP WE NEED?

Yes. Long sleepers have a physiological need for nine or ten hours of sleep, while five hours is enough for short sleepers to wake up refreshed.

IS SLEEPWALKING A SLEEP DISORDER?

Yes; it is a parasomnia. Although it does not really affect the sufferer's sleep quality, it can be dangerous for the sleepwalker, as they are not aware of their movements.

IS IT TRUE THAT THE OLDER WE GET, THE LESS SLEEP WE NEED?

No; our sleep needs do not change as we age. What changes is the way our sleep is organised: we spend less time in deep sleep and REM sleep, while we spend longer in phase I sleep. This means that older people need to take short naps throughout the day.

IS IT TRUE THAT ANY SLEEP WE GET BEFORE MIDNIGHT IS TWICE AS RESTFUL?

No. The first three hours of sleep are the most restorative because this is when we sleep most deeply, but this is not affected by the time we go to bed.

WHAT IS THE OPTIMAL SLEEPING POSITION?

Any position is good; there is no specific position that encourages good-quality sleep. It is a matter of personal choice: you should opt for the most comfortable position for you.

AM I DOING THE RIGHT THING BY FOLLOWING SEVERAL DIFFERENT TREATMENTS TO CURE MY SLEEPING PROBLEMS?

Yes, if you are opting for natural treatments or a holistic approach. Nonetheless, a single treatment can be just as effective as following several at once. You should choose which treatment to follow based on the nature of the problem and your personal preferences.

We want to hear from you!
Leave a comment on your online library
and share your favourite books on social media!

FURTHER READING

BIBLIOGRAPHY

- (No date) *Académie Européenne des Médicines Naturelles.* [Online]. [Accessed 22 January 2018]. Available from: <http://www.aemn.org/>

- (No date) *Association Française de Thérapie Comportementale et Cognitive.* [Online]. [Accessed 22 January 2018]. Available from: <http://www.aftcc.org/>

- Angier, N. (1995) Modern Life Suppresses An Ancient Body Rhythm. *The New York Times.* [Online]. [Accessed 22 January 2018]. Available from: <http://www.nytimes.com/1995/03/14/science/modern-life-suppresses-an-ancient-body-rhythm.html?pagewanted=all>

- Anselme, C. (2013) Apprendre à mieux dormir. *Bioinfo.* 127.

- (No date) *Blog Yogamrita.* [Online]. [Accessed 22 January 2018]. Available from: <http://www.yogamrita.com/blog/>

- Chopra, D. (2009) *Bien dormir avec l'ayurveda.* Paris: Dangles.

- Delhamende, M-A. (2013) Les territoires du sommeil. *Agenda Plus.* [Online]. [Accessed 22 January

2018]. Available from: <https://www.agendaplus.
be/index.php/be/publications/dossier/78457/
les-territoires-du-sommeil>

- Ekirch, R. (2005) *At Day's Close: A History of
  Nighttime.* New York: W.W. Norton & Company.

- Ferron, N. (2013) *Bien dormir, c'est malin.* Paris:
  Leduc.s.

- (No date) *France Sophrologie.* [Online]. [Accessed
  22 January 2018]. Available from: <http://www.
  france-sophrologie.com/>

- Freud, M. (2013) *Se réconcilier avec le sommeil.
  40 exercices faciles et efficaces.* Paris: Albin Michel.

- Garet, J-J. (2015) *Le grand livre de l'hypnose et de
  l'autohypnose : pour maigrir, dormir, arrêter de
  stresser...* Paris: Leduc.s.

- Gerault, G. (2010) *Retrouver le sommeil. Le petit
  livre des huiles essentielles.* Paris: Albin Michel.

- Guiditta, A. (2007) Sonno e sogno. *Treccani.*
  [Online]. [Accessed 22 January 2018]. Available
  from: <http://www.treccani.it/enciclopedia/
  sonno-e-sogno_%28Enciclopedia-della-Scien-
  za-e-della-Tecnica%29/>

- Hallépée, D. (2012) *Mon chat m'a dit, mon chien m'a
  dit.* Domptin, France: Carrefour du Net.

- Hegarty, S. (2012) The myth of the eight-hour
  sleep. *BBC.* [Online]. [Accessed 22 January 2018].
  Available from: <http://www.bbc.com/news/

magazine-16964783>

- Houdret, J-C. and de Paillette, I. (2005) *Bien dormir sans se droguer*. Paris: Solar.

- (No date) *Institut Français d'Hypnose*. [Online]. [Accessed 22 January 2018]. Available from: <https://www.hypnose.fr/>

- (No date) *Institut Français d'Hypnose Humaniste & Ericksonienne*. [Online]. [Accessed 22 January 2018]. Available from: <http://www.ifhe.net/>

- (No date) *La Société Française de Recherche et Médecine du Sommeil*. [Online]. [Accessed 22 January 2018]. Available from: <http://www.sfrms.org/>

- Léger, D. (2010) *Le sommeil dans tous ses états*. Paris: Plon.

- (1988) *MacMillan Dictionary for Students*. New York: Simon & Schuster.

- Masson, J-L. (2010) *L'homéopathie de A à Z. Mieux connaître l'homéopathie pour bien l'utiliser au quotidien*. Vanves: Marabout.

- Nocart, C. (2013) Lumière et sommeil : le juste équilibre. *Agenda Plus*. [Online]. [Accessed 22 January 2018]. Available from: <https://www.agendaplus.be/index.php/be/publications/article/alternative-sante/78456/lumiere-et-sommeil--le-juste-equilibre>

- Phyto2000. (No date) *Association des Usagers*

de la Phytothérapie Clinique. [Online]. [Accessed 22 January 2018]. Available from: <http://www.phyto2000.org/>

- Shakespeare, W. (2018) *The Tempest.* CreateSpace Independent Publishing Platform.

- (No date) *Société Belge de Sophrologie et de Relaxation asbl.* [Online]. [Accessed 22 January 2018]. Available from: <http://www.sbsr.be/>

- (No date) *Société Française d'Homéopathie.* [Online]. [Accessed 22 January 2018]. Available from: <http://www.homeopathie-francaise.com/>

- Tran Dinh Can, M. and Jarre, J. (2016) *Comment retrouver toute son énergie.* Monaco: Éditions du Rocher.

- Valnet, J. (1986) *La phytothérapie : se soigner par les plantes.* Paris: Le Livre de Poche.

- Vanopdenbosch, Y. (2013) *La phytothérapie. Se soigner par les plantes médicinales.* Brussels: Amyris.

- Varela, F.J. ed. (1997) *Sleeping, Dreaming and Dying: An Exploration of Consciousness with The Dalai Lama.* Somerville, Massachusetts: Wisdom Publications.

ADDITIONAL SOURCES

- Chopra, D. (2000) *Restful Sleep: The Complete Mind/Body Programme for Overcoming Insomnia.* London: Rider.

- Smayan, V. (2017) *Shiatsu for Inner Harmony and Balance.* Trans. Traynor, C. Brussels: Plurilingua Publishing.

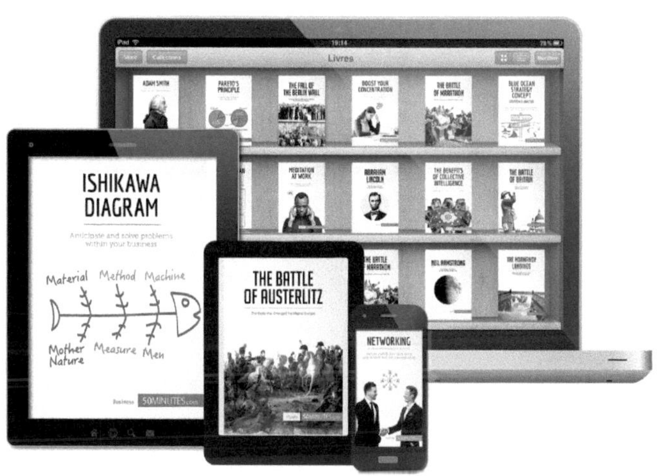
50MINUTES.com
History
Business
Coaching
Book Review
Health & Wellbeing
ISHIKAWA DIAGRAM
Anticipate and solve problems within your business
Material Method Machine
Mother Nature Measure Men
Business 50MINUTES.com
THE BATTLE OF AUSTERLITZ
NETWORKING
IMPROVE YOUR GENERAL KNOWLEDGE
IN A BLINK OF AN EYE !
www.50minutes.com